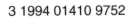

"This entertaining and practical workbook encourages children to follow their natural urge to explore and experiment in order to discover how they experience their world through their senses and to master the feelings that result. As parents work on the exercises with their children, they will find that they understand their children in new ways and perhaps themselves better, as well. In our too-loud, too-bright, too-hurried world, understanding our sensory responses and learning to protect ourselves from overstimulation are important skills for children with special sensory processing challenges, and for the rest of us too."

—Joshua Sparrow, MD, Brazelton Touchpoints Center at Children's Hospital Boston

"The Auers have used their expertise in helping special needs kids to bring us a truly useful work brimming with practical exercises and worksheets that teachers, parents, and especially children can use immediately to better their lives. I can think of few people who work with children in any capacity who couldn't use this book."

—Jeff Stimpson, author of *Alex: The Fathering of a Preemie* and *Alex the Boy: Episodes From A Family's Life With Autism*

"'Sensations That Drive You Nuts!' is a sample of the simple language used in this workbook to help children, their families, and teachers understand sensory processing disorder (SPD). Encouraging children to draw how they feel, recognizing that recess can help one do better in school, becoming a self advocate and helping others when they are in need are some of the many wonderful examples the authors provide."

—Diana A. Henry, MS, OTR/L, FAOTA, author of the Sensory Tools books and DVDs and coauthor of *The Sensory Processing Measures*

Making Sense of Your Senses

A Workbook for Children with Sensory Processing Disorder

CHRISTOPHER R. AUER, MA
MICHELLE M. AUER, MS, OTR

Instant Help Books
A Division of New Harbinger Publications, Inc.

Distributed in Canada by Raincoast Books

Copyright © 2010 by Christopher R. Auer and Michelle M. Auer
          Instant Help Books
          A Division of New Harbinger Publications, Inc.
          5674 Shattuck Avenue
          Oakland, CA 94609
          www.newharbinger.com

Cover design by Amy Shoup
Interior illustrations by Julie Olsen
Cover photograph is a model used for illustrative purposes only.

FSC

Mixed Sources

Product group from well-managed
forests and other controlled sources

Cert no. SW-COC-002283
www.fsc.org
© 1996 Forest Stewardship Council

Library of Congress Cataloging-in-Publication Data

Auer, Christopher R.
 Making sense of your senses : a workbook for children with sensory processing disorder / Christopher R. Auer and Michelle M. Auer.
   p. cm.
 ISBN 978-1-57224-836-6 (pbk.) -- ISBN 978-1-57224-837-3 (pdf ebook)
 1. Sensory integration dysfunction in children--Treatment--Problems, exercises, etc. I. Auer, Michelle M. II. Title.
 RJ496.S44A94 2010
 618.92'8--dc22

                         2010037742

12   11   10

10   9   8   7   6   5   4   3   2   1

First Printing

Contents

A Note to Kids

Dear Reader,

My name is Michelle, and I work with kids at their schools. Many of them say that getting through their school day can be hard. Some kids tell me that noises bother them, that they have a hard time sitting or writing, or that they need more space. Others feel that they need to squeeze something, stretch, or move around in order to pay attention. I love it when I can teach them ways to enjoy being a kid.

My husband's name is Chris. He works with teachers, parents, and people who want to be teachers. He does many of the same things at work as I do, except he spends more time with adults who work with children.

We are also parents. Of our three children, one has some of the same challenges at school as the children I work with. At home, he doesn't like certain smells. He hates the feel of certain clothes and thinks it's torture to get a haircut. He has a hard time sleeping unless his bed is just right. He's also smart and funny, and he loves riding his bike.

Your parent or some other adult who cares about you thinks that your reactions to touching, tasting, smelling, hearing, and seeing make your life difficult. That's where this book comes in. By working through the activities, we hope you'll have fun, learn some ways to make life easier, and "make sense of your senses." We believe that with some practice, you'll start to feel better—and life will get just a little bit easier. Who knows—you might even be able to help someone else with the new skills you'll learn in this workbook!

A Note to Parents

Some people like spicy foods; others don't. Some like vanilla; others prefer chocolate. How we interpret sensory information—through touching, tasting, smelling, hearing, and seeing—is what makes each of us unique.

Our ability to make sense of this information allows us to learn, to avoid hazards, and to experience pleasure. Approximately 5–10 percent of people interpret sensory information differently than most of the population. Light touch may arouse panic in one person, while someone at the other end of that spectrum may appear not to feel any sort of pain at all. When responses, or the lack of responses, to sensory information significantly interfere with daily living, the person may have what is known as sensory processing disorder (SPD).

This workbook was written to help children with SPD. Some children with attention-deficit/hyperactivity disorder (ADHD), autism, and other developmental conditions have SPD coexisting with or underlying these diagnoses. Regardless of the cause, the symptoms of SPD can have a serious impact on the functioning of a child and the entire family.

The activities in this book can develop your child's awareness, understanding, and ability to cope with SPD in healthy ways, both at home and at school. Your child can learn to recognize how he responds to different senses and can master self-calming techniques, ways to keep organized, and even strategies to cope with brothers and sisters.

Your child may need your assistance in working through this book. At the least, he will need encouragement to be patient and work at his own pace. When he completes each activity, you can help him celebrate. You can also help by noticing and rewarding efforts to use new skills throughout the day. We hope your child will have fun while learning.

As parents of a child with ADHD and SPD, we know the challenges can be great, but there are many reasons to be hopeful. In overcoming one challenge in life, whether it be coping with loud noises or going to the dentist, your child may realize that others can be conquered as well. That's an important lesson to learn and one that will help for years to come.

Sincerely,

Christopher R. Auer, MA
Michelle M. Auer, MS OTR

For You to Know

Learning new skills can be a lot of fun and make your life better. It takes effort, and it's not always easy, but having a reward to look forward to along the way can help it seem easier.

Do you remember what it was like when you learned to ride a bike? Perhaps at first you got frustrated and angry. You may have cried or fallen or gotten scrapes and bruises, but eventually you learned how to coast by yourself. Now you probably love to ride around your neighborhood on your own.

Just like riding a bike, learning new skills can be really exciting. Imagine what it would be like without things bothering you all the time—things like noises, smells, eating at the table, or getting dressed. With a little hard work, it's possible.

For You to Do

Read the list below and put a check mark next to each reward you'd like to earn. Then go back and rank those you've marked. Use "1" for something that's really, really great and "5" for something that's just okay. This ranking will help you and your parent develop a plan for earning and receiving rewards.

There might be other things you'd like that aren't listed. That's fine. We've left some room for your own ideas.

- ☐ Playing a game
- ☐ Inviting a friend over
- ☐ Using the computer
- ☐ Special time with your mom or dad
- ☐ A special snack (list it here) _____
- ☐ Going to the movies
- ☐ A new toy (list it here) _____
- ☐ Going swimming
- ☐ Going to the park
- ☐ New clothes
- ☐ Money
- ☐ A sleepover
- ☐ Ice cream
- ☐ Staying up late
- ☐ A favorite activity with the family (list it here) _____
- ☐ Going to your favorite restaurant (list it here) _____
- ☐ Going fishing

- ☐ Making cookies
- ☐ A new game
- ☐ Riding your bike
- ☐ New art supplies
- ☐ A new book
- ☐ Making a fort
- ☐ Going bowling
- ☐ Favorite foods (list three here) _____
- ☐ Playing outside
- ☐ A playdate with friend(s)
- ☐ Your own idea (list it here) _____
- ☐ Your own idea (list it here) _____

... *And More to Do*

Ask your parent to help you work out a plan for how you will earn the rewards you want. For example, will you get a reward for every activity you complete in this book, or do you need to complete a few to get a bigger reward? Also, think of one big reward that you'd like to earn for completing all the activities. Maybe you'd like to have a party with a group of your friends or get a new toy or game. Whatever you decide, the real reward you'll have from working through these activities is more fun—at home and at school. That's worth working for, isn't it?

Reward   **What I Need to Accomplish**

_____   _____

_____   _____

_____   _____

_____   _____

_____   _____

The BIG Reward

_____

What I Need to Do to Earn the BIG Reward

_____

_____

For You to Know

You can have many different feelings inside your body; for example, you may feel happy, sad, angry, frustrated, or frightened. Things happening outside your body, such as temperature, wind, noise, or the level of activity around you, can affect these feelings. It's important to understand your feelings so that you know how to take care of yourself.

Madison opened the door and stepped into the hot sun with her bathing suit and sandals on. She was all set for swimming. She took a few steps toward the pool. Squeak, squish, squeak, squish—gum on the bottom of her sandals! She hated the feel of the gum sticking to the concrete. She took a few more steps—splash! Her brother threw a bucket of water on her. Stinging drops of cold water ran down her back. The gum on her sandals, the cold streaks down her back, and her annoying brother were too much. Madison ran back inside—squeak, squish, squeak, squish—crying all the way.

For You to Do

When things around you become overwhelming, you may have lots of different feelings. And having lots of feelings can make you feel even more overwhelmed—like things are just too much to handle. Some of the words people use to describe feelings are

happy	sad	angry	lonely	frustrated	shy
excited	guilty	nervous	scared	surprised	disappointed
curious	afraid	calm	joyful	brave	embarrassed

Circle the feeling you like the best and think of a time you recently experienced it. Now underline a feeling you don't like having and think of a time you recently experienced it.

In the boxes below, write the name of the feeling you like and the one you don't like. Draw a picture of what you were doing when you experienced each of these feelings.

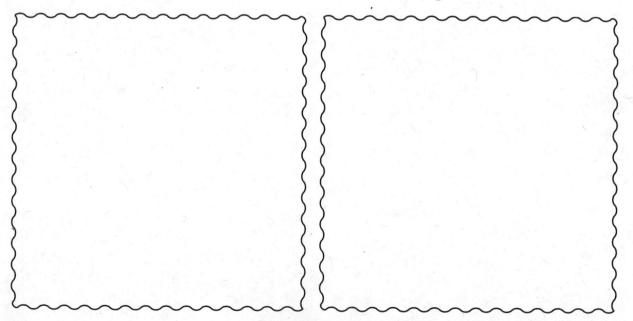

Feeling I Like   *Feeling I Don't Like*

... And More to Do

It's important to learn how to identify what you're feeling as you experience things. Once you can name your feelings, it's easier to express them and decide what you need to do to take care of yourself.

Try to guess how Madison may have felt in each of these situations.

Madison stepped into the hot sun with her bathing suit and sandals on.

Feeling: _____

She got gum on the bottom of her sandals.

Feeling: _____

Her brother splashed her.

Feeling: _____

Stinging drops of cold water ran down her back.

Feeling: _____

What do you think Madison could do to feel better after leaving the pool? Write some advice you would give her so that she can enjoy the rest of her day.

_____

_____

_____

Activity 3

Your Senses Help You Make Choices

For You to Know

Your senses of touch, taste, smell, hearing, and sight help you understand the world around you and make choices about what you like or don't like.

To Janaldo, spaghetti sauce looks and smells like green sewer slime about to take over the world. It's not his fault; his senses just tell him that he does not like spaghetti sauce.

Your senses are involved in choosing things you like or don't like. For example, if you were handed garlic-flavored ice cream, you might be more hesitant the next time someone offered you ice cream. On the other hand, you might be happy to go to the park if it had been a nice, warm day the last time you were there and you had a great time playing with your friends.

Making Sense of Your Senses

For You to Do

In each space below, draw one of your favorite activities; for example, you might like playing with friends, reading, riding your bike, or hanging out with your dog. You don't have to be a good artist. As you draw, think about all the senses that are involved in doing each activity—what does it sound like, look like, smell like, and taste like? How does it feel? On the blank lines, tell why you choose to do each activity.

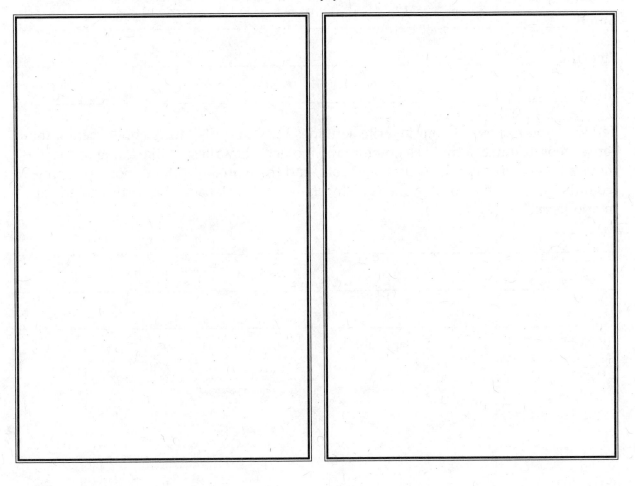

_____

_____

_____

... And More to Do

Look at one of your drawings. Are any of your senses involved? Describe how.

Touch _____

Taste _____

Smell _____

Hearing _____

Sight _____

Tell why you like one of your favorite activities. As you write, think about each of the senses. For example, John likes going to the movies. He writes: "I like going to the movies because the theater is dark and cool, and there are lots of loud noises coming from the screen. I like to sit in the squishy chairs and rock back and forth while I eat my popcorn."

_____

_____

_____

For You to Know

When your senses of taste and touch work well, they can keep you from getting hurt or eating something that might make you sick. They can also make you feel good, like when you get a big hug, sleep in a snuggly bed, or enjoy a delicious treat.

When your senses don't work quite right, things you need to do, like getting dressed, taking a bath, getting a haircut, or having your nails cut, might seem awful. You might also have a hard time doing things that other kids enjoy, like going swimming, trying different foods, or playing in the yard.

Or maybe you're the kind of kid who wants to touch everything you see—people around you, things in the store, or all the furniture in the room. That might bother your friends, and things can get broken.

Maybe your senses of taste and touch don't work like other people's do. But that doesn't mean you can't have fun with your senses by learning more about them.

For You to Do

Taste

First, ask your parent if you can use some foods from your kitchen to do an experiment. You'll probably need to agree to clean up any mess. Once you get the okay, your job is to choose three foods:

- One food you know you really like a lot

- A second food you don't especially like or dislike but are okay with

- A third one you don't like very much at all (but not something that will make you sick)

The foods you choose can be something you drink or eat. Which foods did you choose? Write them here in the space that matches:

Like _____

Okay with _____

Dislike _____

Now follow these steps:

1. Prepare the three foods so that you can take just small bites. Place each on a paper plate on the table.

2. This next part works best if you can't see the foods, so try to keep your eyes closed. If that sounds too scary, you could ask a parent to stay with you. Shuffle the plates around.

3. With your eyes closed (if you can), choose one of the foods, and put a bite into your mouth. Notice what the food feels like in your mouth. Do you like it? How does it taste? Is it sweet, sour (like lemons), or salty?

Write a few words about what you were thinking when you tried the samples.

When I tasted the food I usually like, _____

_____

When I tasted the food I'm usually okay with eating, _____

_____

When I tasted the food I usually dislike, _____

_____

Touch

This time, you're going to experience the sense of touch. Look around your house and gather three things: one you think you would like to touch because it would feel good, one you think would be just okay to touch, and one you think you would dislike touching. Try to be adventurous in your choices, and again, try not to make a mess during your search.

What three things did you find? List them here:

Like _____

Okay with _____

Dislike _____

Now it's time to have some fun. Put each object in a box or in a bowl in front of you on the table. Without looking, shuffle the objects around on the table. Reach your hand in and … touch.

What did the object feel like? Did it feel soft, squishy, wet, or pointy? Did you want to pull your hand away or did you want to feel more?

Write a few words about what you were thinking as you touched each object.

When I touched the object I thought would feel good, _____

_____

When I touched the object I thought would feel okay, _____

_____

When I touched the object I thought I would dislike touching, _____

_____

... And More to Do

Think about what it was it like for you to do this activity. Maybe you discovered that you feel really strongly about certain tastes and things you touch. Are there things that bother you? If so, list them here:

_____ _____ _____

_____ _____ _____

Are there things you can taste and touch that you really like? If so, list them here:

_____ _____ _____

_____ _____ _____

Finally, look at the lists you just wrote. Do you see anything similar about the items on the "don't like" list? Do you see anything similar about the items on the "like" list? Write down your thoughts.

_____

_____

_____

For You to Know

Being able to smell helps keep you healthy and safe. Your nose can tell you when a pan is burning or when food is rotten. It can even tell you when your brother needs to take a bath and wash his feet!

Some kids have noses that work too much. Lots of things smell bad. When everything smells bad, it can be hard to find anything that seems good to eat. It might also be hard to sit in the school cafeteria or other places where food is being prepared.

For You to Do

Find ten things to smell. Choose some things you think you will like and some things you think will take lots of courage to smell. Just don't pick anything really gross. You may want to try salad dressings, spices, fruit, garlic, bread, deodorant, leaves, flowers, shoes, and maybe … dirty socks.

Now smell each of your items. After your nose has done its job, line up your items on a table from best smelling to the absolute worst. Write them below, with the best-smelling thing listed first.

My Ten Smelly Things

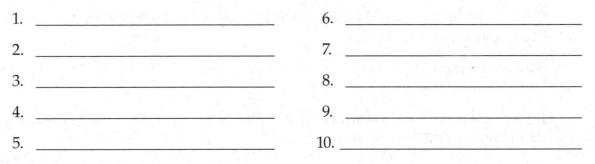

1. _____   6. _____

2. _____   7. _____

3. _____   8. _____

4. _____   9. _____

5. _____   10. _____

What was your best-smelling thing? When you smelled it, what were you thinking? How did you feel?

_____

_____

_____

What was your worst-smelling thing? How did you feel when you smelled it? What was this experience like for you?

_____

_____

_____

... And More to Do

Smells can make you feel great or awful. When you know what smells bother you the most, you can try to avoid them. Can you think of any things that you really can't stand the smell of, either at home or at school? If so, list them here:

_____

_____

Sometimes you may not be able to avoid smells that bother you. When that happens, you might try these ideas:

- Carry some lip balm that is scented with a smell you like. Put it on your lips, or even right under your nose.

- Squeeze your hands and curl your toes—hard. Sometimes it helps to focus your body on another sense.

- If there are people around who might be able to help get rid of the smell, let them know it's bothering you.

- If all else fails, keep some tissues in your pocket and cover your nose.

> ## For You to Know
>
> Sounds can shape how you feel. Some, like music or laughter, can help you feel calm or happy. Other sounds may be annoying or even hurt your ears. For some kids, lots of noises bother them—especially loud ones. Some kids get so mad that noise makes it hard for them to focus on what they're doing.

Tick, tick, tick … Sam looked at the clock on the wall and wished he could throw his math book at it. Tick, tick, tick … He stared down at the problems he was supposed to be doing, but the noise from that stupid clock kept him from being able to concentrate. Sam started to feel angry. His fingers were gripped around his pencil. His body was tense.

Next to him, Alyssa started to sniffle. She had come to school with a cold. Sniff, sniff, cough, sno-o-o-ort … Sam pressed down so hard on his pencil that its point broke.

For You to Do

In this activity, you're going to be a noise detective. You're going to sit and listen (and take some notes). You can listen in your home, in the yard, at school—anyplace that you enjoy. You'll need a notebook, a pen, and a timer.

When you are ready, set the timer for ten minutes and start listening. Write down each noise you hear and how you feel when you hear that noise. To help, we've listed some feeling words you might use:

Happy—safe, calm, joyful, peaceful, relaxed, content

Sad—awful, lonely, down, blue, rotten, disappointed

Mad—irritated, annoyed, angry, frustrated, grouchy, cranky

Afraid—worried, startled, nervous, tense, scared

What I Hear	How I Feel
_____	_____
_____	_____
_____	_____
_____	_____
_____	_____
_____	_____
_____	_____
_____	_____

Were there any noises that you really liked or any that really bothered you? Write them down.

_____

Do the noises you liked have anything in common? Tell what.

_____

Do the noises you disliked have anything in common? Tell what.

_____

... And More to Do

Do short, sharp noises bother you a lot? Do low, constant noises make you uncomfortable? If you know which noises bother you the most, you can make plans to help yourself the next time you hear them.

Here are some tricks you can try when you can't stop or get away from a noise that bothers you:

- Use earplugs.

- Hum a favorite song to yourself.

- Cover your ears.

- Think of something other than the noise—maybe something funny or a favorite holiday or something you're looking forward to.

For You to Know

Even when they're looking at the same object or event, two people may notice different things. They may also have very different feelings about what they're seeing.

"That girl tripped Tara!" said Megan.

"She did not," said Janaya.

"Janaya, weren't you watching? Number 3 stuck her leg out just to trip Tara so she wouldn't score a goal."

"I was watching and Tara just fell down," said Janaya. "Number 3 was like four feet away. There's no way she could have tripped Tara."

"I think the bright sun is making you dizzy. I'm telling you, Janaya, it was a trip," said Megan.

"Well, the sun and all the people moving around *are* making me dizzy, but I think you're the one who needs some big, thick glasses—you know, the ones that weigh about ten pounds!" said Janaya.

For You to Do

You get to watch a movie! Well, at least for about fifteen seconds. Choose your favorite movie and fast-forward to a good scene. (With a parent's permission, a short online clip would work well too.) When you're ready, you're going to watch for only ten to fifteen seconds. During this time, see how much you can notice—people, clothes, colors, and other details. On the lines that follow, write what you noticed. If you prefer to draw, draw everything you noticed in the box.

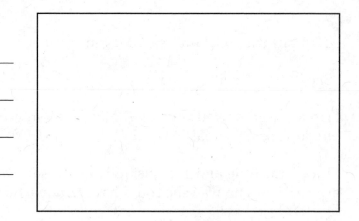

Now watch the scene again. Were there any details you missed? What were they?

It can be fun to have others watch the same scene to see what they notice. Ask your parent, friend, brother, or sister do this activity and compare what each noticed with your observations. Were there any differences? What were they?

... *And More to Do*

Just like people are different in what they notice, some people have different feelings in reaction to what they see. Some people feel sick when they see things moving really quickly. Some people react strongly to bright or flickering light. Are there things that bother you when you see them? If so, what are they?

_____

_____

_____

You can experiment to make what's around you more pleasing to your eyes. When you like to see what's around you, you may feel better. These ideas can be fun to try:

- Wear sunglasses or a baseball hat to block out the bright sun from your eyes.

- Make some pictures (or other type of art) and display them in your room.

- Keep your room clean at home and your desk clean at school.

- Turn off some of the lights in your room.

- Look at different colors (in a magazine or at a store) and notice which ones make you feel calm. See if your parent will get you some sheets for your bed and covers for your schoolbooks with those colors.

For You to Know

Some kids react very strongly to particular sensations. If you can notice what things bother you the most, you may be able to avoid them or make a plan for how to deal with them.

"*Yuck*! Get that away!" Jackson pushed his bowl of food across the table. "I hate the smell of garlic!" He sat back in his seat, on the verge of tears. His shirt was pulled up over his nose as a defense against any remaining garlic fumes still lurking around.

His sister sucked a noodle into her mouth—sluuurrp! She stared at him with half a noodle dangling from her lips. To Jackson, it looked like a captured worm.

"Disgusting!" Jackson cried out. "That's so gross!"

Tears started running. He felt betrayed. He thought everyone knew that he hated the smell of garlic and looking at stringy noodles.

Sensations That Drive You Nuts! Activity 8

For You to Do

With a parent's permission, look through old magazines or search the Internet and find pictures of things that drive you crazy. Cut out or print out the pictures and paste them into the box below. As you do, think about how the thing in each picture makes you feel and what you don't like about it.

... And More to Do

Look back at your pictures. How many pictures do you have that go along with

taste? _____ touch? _____ smell? _____ hearing? _____ sight?

Which sense do you have the most pictures for? _____

Which do you have the least for? _____

How do your answers match your feelings about each of these senses? For example, if you have the most pictures of things that you don't like the taste of, is that the sense that bothers you the most?

_____

_____

Describe one or two things that really irritate you. For example, do you dislike the feel of foam so much that you'd rather eat a raw onion, smell a dirty sock, and listen to a loud motorcycle than have to even touch the foam with the tip of your baby finger?

_____

_____

Pick one picture that shows a sensation you recently encountered. Tell what happened.

_____

_____

Are you usually able to avoid this sensation? If not, what do you do when it comes your way?

_____

_____

Share your collage and your answers with your parent, and explain how you feel when you encounter each of these sensations.

For You to Know

When your senses don't work as they should, it can be difficult to get things done throughout your day. All of your senses need to work together so that your brain can get the right information to tell your body what to do.

"What are you cutting?" asked Emma.

"I'm making a snowflake to go along with my story," replied Joshua.

Emma looked at his paper and said, "That doesn't look like a snowflake at all."

Joshua held the folded paper in his hand. It looked like his dog had tried to eat his homework. Bits of paper were torn off.

Joshua hated to cut things. Sometimes he would drop the scissors, the paper, or both. And even if he didn't drop anything, he usually ended up ripping the paper. No matter how closely he watched what he was doing, it was like his hands didn't work.

For You to Do

You're going to do some experiments that will make your senses not work as well as they should. As you do these experiments, notice what you are thinking and feeling.

Touch

Ask your parent for some rubber gloves. If you don't have any rubber gloves, you can use mittens, wool gloves, or even a towel covering your hands. Once you've got your hands covered, grab a pencil and try writing or typing a short note to a friend.

What was this like for you? _____

_____

Taste

Eat a saltine cracker (or something else that doesn't have much flavor) and then try something you really like to eat.

What was this like for you? _____

_____

Smell

Put a bit of deodorant or perfume under your nose. Then try smelling different foods you have in your refrigerator or pantry.

What was this like for you? _____

_____

Hearing

Turn on the TV to a show you like or turn on some good music. Grab two washcloths and hold them up tight against your ears. With your ears covered, try listening to your show or music for a minute or two.

What was this like for you? _____

_____

Sight

Grab a pair of sunglasses (the darker the better) and a book you'd like to read. Now go to a dim room in your house, put on your sunglasses, and try reading a page or two.

What was this like for you? _____

_____

... And More to Do

Think of your favorite thing to do. What would it be like if all of your senses were dulled when you were doing your favorite thing?

_____

_____

Do you wish one of your senses could be stronger? If so, which one? _____

Why do you wish that sense were stronger?

_____

_____

For You to Know

Some kids really like certain sensations. When you know which sensations you like, you can use that information to keep you motivated when things are hard.

"Stop eating with your fingers!" said Joe's mom. Every night Joe got yelled at for picking at his food with his fingers. He found it hard to eat noodles with a fork. Mostly though, it felt good to squish the noodles between his fingers. He liked the warmth. It was also fun to roll the noodles into a ball and then eat them. And, he had to admit, it was sort of fun to drive his mom crazy.

For You to Do

With your parent's permission, print out pictures from the Internet of things you love to touch, taste, smell, hear, and see, or cut them out from old magazines. Paste these pictures below.

... And More to Do

Look back at your pictures. How many pictures do you have that go along with

taste? _____ touch? _____ smell? _____ hearing? _____ sight?

Which sense do you have the most pictures for? _____

You can add things to your room or surroundings that will allow you to experience sensations related to that sense. For example, Victoria generally liked to touch things. In her room, she kept a box of sand to play with, some small balls to roll around in her hands, and a squishy ball that she could squeeze while reading.

Are there things related to your favorite sense that you'd like to have in your room? They should be realistic—no freezer full of ice cream next to your bed! Write some of these things here:

_____

_____

_____

For You to Know

You can help yourself become better at sports by practicing your skills. When you improve your playing, it's likely that you'll enjoy sports more.

The best athletes work hard and spend years learning their sport. They know where they are strong and where they need to practice more. For example, soccer players may take ballet lessons to strengthen their legs and become more fit. By trying different activities, they learn more about their bodies.

Athletes also need to have a good sense of coordination. Coordination is the ability to tell where parts of your body are located relative to your surroundings, and relative to each other. It can help you to move yourself or other objects. It is a result of sensations from your skin and muscles and also from your sense of balance.

For You to Do

This activity offers two choices to challenge your sense of coordination. The first choice will require some materials and some construction that you'll need a parent's help for. There's no construction involved in the second choice, but it would still be a good idea to have a parent help to make sure you don't fall.

Choice 1

You will need two empty metal coffee cans, some twine, a hammer, a nail, and a parent to help.

Turn one coffee can over so the open end is facing toward the ground. Have your parent use the hammer and the nail to punch a hole on one side of the can and another on the opposite side, each about an inch down from the closed end. Repeat with the other can.

Thread the twine through one of the holes, across the inside of the can, and out the other hole. Pull enough twine to make a loop large enough so that you can stand on top of the can and hold the loop comfortably with your hand. Cut the twine, and tie the end of the loop. Repeat with the other can.

On a steady surface and away from any obstacles (in case you fall), stand on both cans while holding the twine loops. Now try walking while keeping your feet on the cans. See if you can walk forward and then turn around, all while keeping your feet on the cans.

Choice 2

You will need a pair of high-heeled shoes and your mom's permission to use them. You may want a soccer ball, or another ball that you can kick.

On a clear, level area away from any obstacles, step into those high-heeled shoes. Once you have your balance, see if you can walk around. If you can walk around safely and you're feeling confident, see if you can kick the ball. Be careful not to fall!

... And More to Do

What was this activity like for you?

_____

_____

_____

It usually takes lots of practice to become comfortable at doing new things. If this activity was difficult, it may mean that your body was asked to do something it hasn't done before. That's okay. You can practice and get better.

What physical activities do you think you're good at?

_____

_____

_____

What physical activities would you like to be better at?

_____

_____

_____

Making Sense of Your Senses

For You to Know

Your muscles and joints tell your body if you are using too much or too little pressure to do things. By doing activities to work your muscles and joints, you'll feel more relaxed, and you'll be more aware of what your body is telling you.

Sofia had just broken another pencil while writing at her desk. "Why do you always do things so hard?" Kyle asked. "You don't have to squeeze the pencil that way! It's not going to run away."

"Yeah, and when we play tag, you don't have to push!" added Ava.

At home, Sofia got in trouble for jumping onto the couches, for slamming the refrigerator door, and for gripping her fork like she was trying to bend it into some form of weaponry (so said her dad).

Most of the time, Sofia didn't know that she was being rough—except when she was jumping and crashing onto the couches. She knew that was against the rules of her house, but after she jumped and crashed, she felt better and more relaxed.

For You to Do

In this activity, you are going to make an obstacle course. Depending on where you live and the time of the year, it can be inside or outside. The first step is to decide on a location. It should be free of anything that might hurt you or break.

Once you've decided on a location, look around the house or yard for obstacles—things you have to go over, around, or through on your race from one end of the course to the other. It might help to plan your course by making a drawing of what obstacles you'd like to use, where they will be, and the route you will take through your course. Make your drawing in the space below. Show your drawing to your parent to make sure your plan is okay. Once you have the okay, go for it!

... And More to Do

What was the experience of doing your obstacle course like?

_____

_____

_____

How did you feel afterward?

_____

_____

How can you change your course to make it more challenging?

_____

_____

For You to Know

Tuning in on what is happening around you is a good way to learn about your body and your senses. It can also help you be more focused and calm.

After lunch, Alexis and the other kids in her class went back their classroom and sat at their desks. This was quiet time. Alexis laid her head on her desk and closed her eyes. She heard the air conditioning pumping out cool air into the room. She listened for other sounds. Other classes were still playing outside, and she could hear kids calling out and laughing. The fish tank was humming away, sending water through the filter. The principal was talking to a student in the hall.

Alexis focused only on the sound of her own breathing and the feel of her lungs taking in and letting out air. When the lights came on, she felt rested and ready for the afternoon's work.

For You to Do

For this activity, you will need a timer. Your task is to find a quiet place in your house or outside where you can sit comfortably. When you are ready, set the timer for one minute, and then close your eyes.

While your eyes are closed, focus on each of your senses. Ask yourself

1. What do I feel around me?

2. What do I smell?

3. What do I taste?

4. What do I hear?

5. What was the last thing I saw before I closed my eyes?

If you can't remember each of these five questions, that's okay. Just be aware of what you are sensing around you. When the timer goes off, open your eyes and be aware of the first thing you see.

... And More to Do

What was this experience like for you?

_____

_____

_____

What sense were you most aware of? _____

Would this activity be helpful for you to do every day? Why or why not?

_____

_____

_____

For You to Know

Coordination and balance are important for sports and also for games you might want to play with your friends on the playground or in the neighborhood—like capture the flag or catch—or for just running around having fun. You can improve your level of coordination and balance through regular practice in fun activities.

"Everyone move up!" called Taylor. "If Abigail kicks the ball, it's not going to go far."

Abigail looked directly at Taylor. She was determined to kick the ball way out into the field, or maybe right toward Taylor.

Taylor rolled the ball. Abigail positioned herself for what was going to be the hardest kick of her life. Boom! She tried to kick so hard that she missed and fell flat on the ground. Everyone was laughing, except Abigail.

On the way home, she practiced kicking small rocks that were in her path on the sidewalk. She even practiced balancing on the curb. Later that evening, she practiced kicking a ball against a wall. She was determined to get better.

For You to Do

You are going to decide on five exercises and then try to do them every day for one week. To get you started, we've suggested five exercises. Try to think of five more, and write them in the chart below.

Now circle the five exercises you want to try. They can be the five we suggested, the five you thought of, or any combination. Try to do them every day. Use the chart to track your progress. Each day, put a check mark in the box next to all the exercises you did that day.

Activity	M	T	W	TH	F	SA	S
Do ten sit-ups.							
Walk across the room on your tiptoes.							
Walk across the room on your heels.							
Toss a ball up in the air and catch it ten times.							
Kick a ball toward a wall. With one foot, stop the ball after it bounces off the wall. Do this ten times.							

... And More to Do

What do you think your level of balance and coordination was at the beginning of the week? Rate it from 1 to 5.

1	2	3	4	5
(poor)		(fair)		(great)

What do you think your level of balance and coordination is now? Rate it from 1 to 5.

1	2	3	4	5
(poor)		(fair)		(great)

Do you think you improved? If so, try continuing this plan, but every week change your routine by adding new activities or making the existing activities a bit more challenging. If you don't think you improved, try the plan for another week with the same activities. Stick to it!

For You to Know

It can be very tempting to slump in your seat and forget about your body and your surroundings. But kids who sit up and stand straight usually look more alert and confident. When you look confident, chances are you will feel confident too!

Hannah was slumped over the dinner table. "Hannah, you look like you're falling asleep. Can you please sit up!" ordered her mother. Hannah's mom was always telling her to sit up or stand up straight. As Hannah thought more about her mom's complaint, she realized that her mom was probably right. She looked and felt tired a lot of the time.

For You to Do

One way to look more alert and confident is to wake up your body through your senses. In this activity, you're going to think of lots of different ways to wake yourself up! We've listed some ideas to get you started. Your job is to fill in the spaces with more ideas that you'd like to try. Look at the things around you at home and school. What might alert each of your senses?

If you have a hard time coming up with ideas, you can always experiment. How do you feel if you drink some cold water? How do you feel if you rub a towel on your arms and legs? Try squeezing your hands together. Now try curling your toes.

Sight	Hearing	Smell	Touch	Taste
Take a walk outside.	Listen to music.	Smell a lemon.	Chew on ice.	Put a drop of lemon juice on your tongue.
Turn on the lights.	See how many different sounds you can hear right where you are.		Sit on a bouncy ball.	
			Splash cold water on your face.	

A Workbook for Children with Sensory Processing Disorder

... *And More to Do*

Another way to look more alert and confident is to build up the muscles in your stomach and back. This takes some effort, but you'll look better and feel better. We've listed some ways to help build your muscles. Put a check mark next to those ideas you'd like to try, and then list a few of your own ideas.

- ☐ Swing on a swing.

- ☐ Hop on one foot.

- ☐ Jump rope.

- ☐ Stretch on a bouncy ball.

- ☐ Do a crab walk across the room. (Put your hands and feet on the floor, with your stomach facing the ceiling.)

- ☐ Do the limbo.

- ☐ Stretch your hands toward the sky.

- ☐ Play tug-of-war with a friend or parent.

Kayla got into the backseat of the car with her friend Danielle. Danielle's mom was driving her home from school. "This is the smallest car I've ever been in!" she thought. There were some boxes on the floor so she could hardly move her legs. Even without the boxes, there wasn't much room. She felt like the front seat was in her lap.

"How are you, Kayla?" Danielle's mom asked. Kayla had a hard time answering; she felt like she was about to choke on the smell of perfume that had filled the car. She hadn't noticed it when she first stepped in, but now it was like a cloud that she couldn't get away from.

"Do you two want to listen to some music?" Without waiting for an answer, Danielle's mom turned on some loud music, maybe from the 1970s. Kayla felt like she was going to panic. She felt trapped.

When You're in Tough Spots

For You to Do

Do you remember a time when you were bothered by something and couldn't get away? In the space below, draw a picture of what happened. Be sure to show what was bothering you.

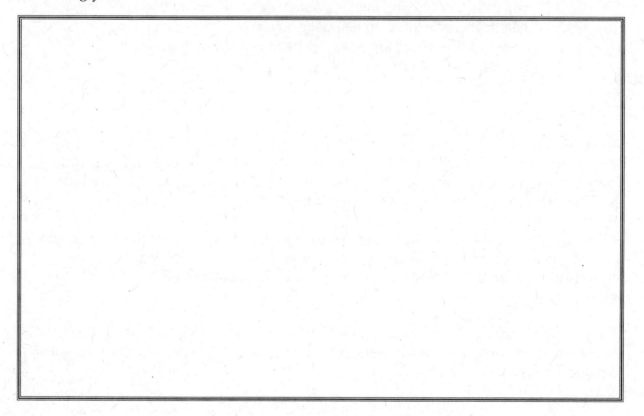

Now that you've finished your drawing, write a couple of sentences to describe what you did to get through the tough spot.

_____

_____

_____

_____

_____

... And More to Do

If you're in a tough spot and things become overwhelming, the first thing to do is to take some deep breaths and see if there's anyone around who can help. If there isn't, try to identify how you feel. Are you feeling hot, sick, angry, or itchy?

We've listed some things that usually help kids. Put a check mark next to each choice that you think you might try in the future. If you can think of your own idea for each sense, write it in the blank space.

If the sense of touch is bothering you, can you

☐ change clothes?

☐ touch something else that feels good?

☐ think of something that makes you happy?

☐ _____

If the sense of taste is bothering you, can you

☐ have a piece of candy or gum in your pocket?

☐ ask for something to drink?

☐ put the bad-tasting object in a napkin?

☐ _____

If the sense of smell is bothering you, can you

☐ put a scarf or sleeve over your nose?

☐ have your parent put a favorite scent on your hand?

☐ put on some good-smelling lip balm?

☐ _____

If the sense of hearing is bothering you, can you

- ☐ use earplugs?
- ☐ listen to something you like, so you don't hear the disturbing noise?
- ☐ focus on a sense that you do like?
- ☐ _____

If the sense of sight is bothering you, can you

- ☐ wear sunglasses?
- ☐ wear a hat?
- ☐ adjust the light?
- ☐ _____

Write a few sentences that describe one or two things you will do to help yourself the next time you are in a tough spot.

_____

_____

_____

_____

_____

For You to Know

Keeping a journal doesn't have to be a lot of work, and it can be a great way to keep track of all the good things that happen. It can also be a way to identify when and why things go wrong, which can help to keep them from happening again. A journal should include significant things that happened, how you felt, what you did, and what you might want to do differently.

"Tell me how your day went," Nick's grandmother said.

"Well, I really liked the pancakes you made this morning. They were yummy," Nick said. "But on the bus to school, I started feeling sick with all the turns. I hate riding the bus."

"So what did you do?" asked his grandmother.

"I remembered what you told me. I opened the window a bit. The air helped. I also focused on curling my toes, over and over. That helped me not think about being sick," Nick answered.

"So what happened when you got to school?"

"Shawn's dad brought in some Jell-O jigglers—you know, the Jell-O stuff you can hold and jiggle? They were great! I loved shaking them, smelling them—they were cherry— and then biting off a piece."

"Was that the best part of your day?" asked his grandmother.

"No, the best part was climbing on the playset with my friends at recess. We played a lot! When we went inside, I felt really relaxed."

"It sounds like you learned some things about yourself, Nick—that opening the window helps you on the bus, that you like Jell-O jigglers, and that playing outside helps you feel relaxed. It would be great for you to write this in your journal, to help you remember. And after you're done, we can make some Jell-O jigglers for dessert!"

A Workbook for Children with Sensory Processing Disorder

For You to Do

In the circle below, draw a simple picture of you. On each of the lines, write a word or two to describe one thing that happened during your day. For example, Nick might write on one of the lines that he ate pancakes. On another, he might write that he rode the bus.

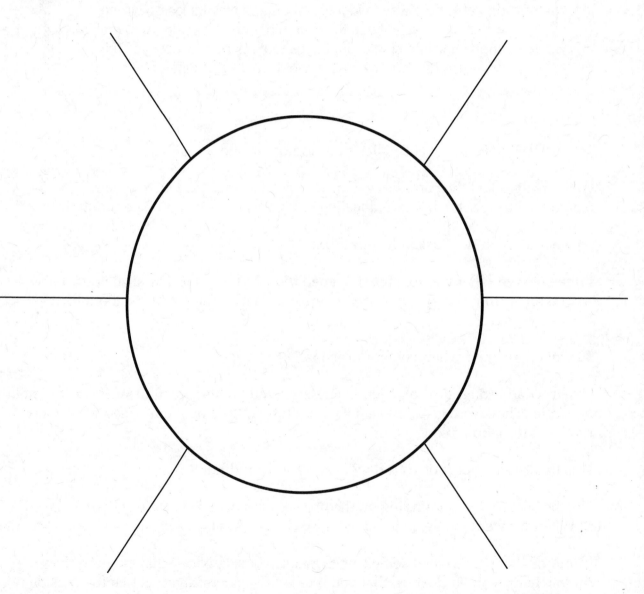

... And More to Do

There are different ways to keep a journal. You can draw or write sentences or fill in a chart like the one here. Look back at what you wrote about your day. From your notes, pick three things that you remember well. Fill in this chart to expand on your thoughts. We've filled in two rows from Nick's day as an example. We encourage you to make some notes every day, so that you can make each new day better.

What happened?	Where were you?	How did you feel?	If what happened wasn't good, what did you do?	What else could you have done?
I started to feel sick.	On the bus	Worried	I curled my toes and opened the window.	Asked to sit in the front
I ate Jell-O jigglers.	School	Happy		

Activity 18   Relaxing After School

For You to Know

When you're relaxed, it's easier to do your homework, get along with the people in your family, and get a good night's sleep. When you get home from school, you can help yourself be more calm and focused by doing fun activities that relax you.

The long bus ride after a day at school usually made Levi feel tense. He could feel the tightness in his jaw and back muscles. He looked up from his game and finally saw his house coming up around the corner. Phew! He jumped off the bus and opened the fence gate.

"Hi Levi," his sitter called as he opened the door. "Come upstairs; I've got your favorite snack."

Levi sat down and crunched on some nuts. As he ate, he could feel his jaw start to relax.

"Let's see how many jumps you can do today," his sitter said when he was finished with his snack.

Levi went downstairs and hopped onto the trampoline. It wasn't big, but it sure was fun. He jumped and jumped, and with every bounce he started to feel better.

After bouncing, he went outside and played in the dirt. That also made him feel better. He liked the coolness of the earth on his hands. Today he was going to dig another tunnel.

For You to Do

In the space below, draw a picture or write some words to describe what you usually do when you get home from school. Include as much detail as you can about your activities.

Look at what you drew or wrote. Which things help you feel more relaxed and focused?

_____

_____

Look at your list of things that help you feel relaxed and focused. Are these quiet, calm activities, or are they active ones that burn energy?

_____

_____

Are these things healthy for your body and your mind? If you think so, tell why.

_____

_____

... And More to Do

With a little imagination, you can find lots of things to do at home to help you be more focused, relaxed, and happy after a long day at school. We've listed some ideas below. If an idea sounds like something you'd like to try either today or tomorrow, put a check mark next to it.

If you like to do active things to relax, you might

- ☐ make a fort
- ☐ jump rope
- ☐ eat something crunchy
- ☐ play in the dirt
- ☐ make an obstacle course
- ☐ play music and dance
- ☐ rake leaves
- ☐ clean your room
- ☐ play with toy cars
- ☐ jump on a trampoline
- ☐ play basketball
- ☐ ride a bike

If you like to do calm things to relax, you might

- ☐ paint
- ☐ draw
- ☐ listen to music
- ☐ snuggle with your pet
- ☐ read
- ☐ go for a walk
- ☐ make a collage
- ☐ take a warm bath

Look back at your list and put a star next to one or two things you'd like to try today or tomorrow when you get home from school. Then try them!

Creating a Calm-Down Space

For You to Know

When things become overwhelming or stressful, it can be helpful to have a place where you can calm down and relax. You can make a space like that for yourself.

"Stop whining! I hate it when you do that!" yelled Rachel. It was 100 degrees outside, and her house didn't have air conditioning.

"Where's my game cartridge?" cried her brother Brett.

"I don't know! Can you just go away! I've got to do my homework, and it's due tomorrow!"

To make things worse, her dad was cooking leftover food on the stove, and it was starting to burn. Rachel hated the smell of burning food.

"Where's my game cartridge? Find it! Help me find it! Please? Where is it?" cried Brett for the fortieth time.

Rachel just wanted to run and hide someplace.

For You to Do

What do you think Rachel was feeling? Write down three feeling words that describe how she may have felt.

_____   _____   _____

Has there ever been a time when things became overwhelming for you? If so, write what was happening when you felt overwhelmed.

_____

_____

What feelings did you have during this situation?

_____

_____

In our family, when people become very upset, we call that having a meltdown. A parent might realize that you're about to have a meltdown, or you might realize it yourself. How can you tell when you're about to have a meltdown?

_____

_____

_____

If you think you're about to have a meltdown, what are some things you can do to take care of yourself? Talk this over with your parent and write down your thoughts.

_____

_____

_____

... And More to Do

With your parent, look around your house for a place where you can go to get away when you feel overwhelmed. You might think of areas behind or between furniture, a closet, a corner in your room, or under the stairs.

Where will you make your calm-down space?

_____

What would you like to put in your calm-down space? We've listed some things grouped by senses to get you thinking, and we've added some blank lines for your own ideas. And please check with your parent before you start setting up your space. Some things may need to be replaced before they get moldy or go into containers so they don't attract critters!

Touch

Pillow, blanket, stuffed animals, squeeze toy, rubber-band ball

_____

_____

Taste

Gum, hard pretzels, nuts, raisins

_____

_____

Smell

Cinnamon stick, vanilla extract on a cotton ball, tea bag, lemon

_____

_____

Hearing

Music player, earplugs, fan, electronic game

_____

_____

Sight

Pictures, trading cards, books, flowers, magazines

_____

_____

For You to Know

If you're calm and relaxed before going to bed, you're more likely to get a good night's sleep and feel refreshed in the morning. Having a bedtime routine and a cozy place to sleep can help.

"I love my bed," Deshawn told his mom as he got ready to sleep. He had the top bunk, and sleeping high up, close to the ceiling, made him feel secure. "When I straighten out all my blankets and crawl under them, I feel like I'm climbing into a cave."

"What about your stuffed animals?" asked his mom.

"Oh, those go all around me, stacked up against the rail. Dinosaur goes by my side, though."

Deshawn climbed the ladder and crawled under the stack of blankets. He took a final look at his army of animals and asked his mom to turn on the fan. He liked the noise and the moving air.

As she left the room, his mom turned on the night-light—not too bright, just enough to see by. Deshawn drifted off to sleep, comfortable and secure.

For You to Do

Think of some things you can do before bed to help you relax. We've listed some ideas for a nightly routine. If you'd like to try an idea, put a check mark next to it. We've added some blank lines for you to write down your own ideas.

- ☐ Read a book.
- ☐ Take a bath.
- ☐ Listen to music.
- ☐ Drink a cup of warm milk.
- ☐ Play with some quiet toys.
- ☐ Draw a picture.
- ☐ Do a puzzle.
- ☐ Put your pajamas in the drier so they're warm for bed.
- ☐ _____
- ☐ _____
- ☐ _____

How can you make your room and your bed a cozy place for sleep? Think of each of your senses and what might feel good. Again, we've listed some ideas to get you thinking. If one sounds good, put a check mark next to it. Write your own ideas on the blank lines.

Touch

- ☐ Lots of blankets
- ☐ Soft pajamas
- ☐ Breeze from a fan
- ☐ Cool sheets
- ☐ _____
- ☐ _____

Smell

- ☐ Newly washed pillowcase
- ☐ Vanilla extract
- ☐ No smell
- ☐ Lavender oil
- ☐ _____
- ☐ _____

Hearing

- ☐ Fan
- ☐ Music
- ☐ Silence
- ☐ _____
- ☐ _____

Sight

- ☐ Night-light
- ☐ Total darkness
- ☐ Lava lamp
- ☐ Flashlight
- ☐ _____
- ☐ _____

Did you notice that the sense of taste isn't included here? That's because eating right before bed can sometimes keep you up, and it's also not good to eat after you've brushed your teeth.

... And More to Do

There are lots of ways to make a cozy, perfect place to sleep. In the space below, draw a picture of how you'd like your room and your bed to be so that you can get the best night's sleep ever.

Activity 21   Getting Ready for School

For You to Know

Kids who have difficulty with their senses often have a harder time getting ready for the day. With some planning, you can help your morning be much more relaxing.

"Wake up!" called Ryan's father. "You have only thirty minutes to get down to the bus stop!"

Ryan felt like he was wearing earmuffs. He couldn't quite hear his dad's words but could tell he was upset. He tried to move, but his body was stiff and heavy. His arms were like weights.

His dad came into his room, barking, "Here, put these clothes on!"

Ryan had somehow made it out of bed, but he was wobbly as he stood. He put on his shirt. "Ouch! Dad, you know I hate tags!" The shirt felt like it was scraping his skin with his every move. When he put on his pants, they felt tight and itchy.

Finally dressed, he made his way to the bathroom, where his dad wet a brush and tried to smooth out his hair. Drops of water ran down Ryan's forehead onto his nose "Stop!" he yelled.

It was too much. Ryan felt stressed and angry. Everything was going wrong—and he was about to miss the bus.

For You to Do

This chart shows some activities kids usually do in the morning, explanations of why they might be hard, and then some ways to make them easier. Add your own and come up with ways to have a better morning by making them easier.

Activity	Why It's Hard	Ways to Make It Easier
Waking up	I don't have any energy.	Have alarm play exciting music. Have a glass of water to drink when I first get out of bed.
Walking to the bathroom	It's scary because it's still dark in the house when I have to wake up.	Have a flashlight by my bed. Keep a light on in the bathroom and a night-light in the hallway.
Getting dressed	I don't like my clothes. They're too tight.	The night before, I will pick out some clothes that I would like to wear to school.

A Workbook for Children with Sensory Processing Disorder

... *And More to Do*

Tell how trying the new things you listed might be able to help you in the morning.

_____

_____

_____

_____

_____

For You to Know

Most kids have homework to do. But when kids mention homework, they usually don't say positive things. With the right environment though, it can be a relaxing experience … well, maybe not relaxing, but certainly less painful.

"I hate doing homework!" Cole complained to his dad.

"What's wrong?" his dad asked.

"I have to do four spelling pages by tomorrow, and I can't concentrate," Cole replied. He was hunched over his little desk in a dark corner of his room. Papers, broken crayons, and pencil shavings covered the surface so that he barely had enough room to work on his packet. He hated writing, too. It was hard for him, and he kept breaking his pencil. And the dog barking across the street didn't help.

"Can't our neighbors take their dog and move?" Cole asked his dad.

For You to Do

At school, if you don't understand how to do an assignment, you probably ask your teacher for help. There might also be other things at your desk or in your classroom to help you. These can be simple things, like a pencil grip, a number line on your desk, or posters around the room to help you with spelling or writing.

What helps you do your work at school? Write some of these things here:

_____

_____

_____

At home, you can try using the same things. It can also help to make the space where you do your homework as pleasing to you as possible. In the circle below, write where you usually do your homework. Then, on each of the lines, write a word to describe this area. Try to think of words that match your senses. What does the area look like? Smell like? Feel like? Sound like?

Making Sense of Your Senses

What do you like about where you do your homework?

_____

_____

_____

What would you like to change about where you do your homework?

_____

_____

_____

... And More to Do

There might be some things you can add to where you do homework to make the experience more enjoyable. We've listed a couple of our favorite things below each sense to get you thinking. You can use the blank lines for your own ideas.

Touch

Pillow behind back, pencil grip, cushion on seat

_____

_____

_____

Taste

Apple juice, celery

_____

_____

_____

Smell

Mint, coffee, bubble gum

_____

_____

_____

Hearing

Soft music, total silence

_____

_____

_____

Sight

Clean area, plant, soft light

_____

_____

_____

Activity 23   Making Mealtimes Easier

For You to Know

A healthy diet can help you have energy for fun things, and it can keep your body in shape. There are so many good foods to try, and with some planning, you can help create some great meals.

"Why did you make spaghetti? I'm going to starve! You know I hate spaghetti," whined Nina.

"Well, that's what's for dinner. If you don't like it, you're welcome to make something yourself. Just be sure to clean up afterward," her mom replied.

Nina opened the refrigerator and pulled her shirt over her nose. She was always afraid of what she might smell. She looked inside and didn't see anything interesting. She looked some more.

"Eggs!" she thought, as she noticed them sitting neatly on the inside of the door. She loved breakfast foods. She saw some tomatoes, cheese, and meat. An omelet! That sounded yummy. She probably needed to add another vegetable though, as she only had tomatoes. Hmmm, what would be good … she hated onions, so that was out. She didn't like anything spicy. Celery! She liked the thought of that. Something crunchy in her meal sounded good.

For You to Do

It might seem hard to eat a healthy diet if you don't like certain textures, tastes, or smells. But there are lots of different kinds of foods, and being able to help plan meals can make things easier.

For this activity, you are going to come up with some meal ideas. There are some rules, though. First, your ideas need to fit the way things are done at your home. So if your parent buys only vegetables or food made from vegetables (but no meat), your ideas should include only vegetables.

To get some ideas of different foods to eat, you can look at supermarket ads on the Internet or in the newspaper. You can also go shopping with your parent and point out foods that look interesting. In the space below, paste pictures, draw, or write the names of some healthy foods that you'd like in a meal.

Next, think about how you would like your meals to be prepared and served. For example, some kids might ask that foods be separated from each other on the plate or that there be no sauces or food that's soft and mushy. If you have any requests, write them here:

_____

_____

_____

... And More to Do

Having some foods that you'd like to try and ideas about their preparation can make meal planning easier for both you and your parent. Use this chart to list your ideas for some meals for the week. Keep in mind that protein foods (like meat, beans, and eggs) are important, but your meals should be mostly vegetables, fruits, and grains, like brown rice.

	Breakfast	Lunch	Dinner
Sunday			
Monday			
Tuesday			
Wednesday			
Thursday			
Friday			
Saturday			

Look over your ideas to make sure that they follow the rules of your house, and change any that don't.

For You to Know

Kids who have problems with their senses sometimes hate haircuts. The reasons can be very different. Some kids feel itchy afterward. Some kids hate the sound of the scissors cutting. And some kids are just afraid of getting a bad haircut!

Matthew's mom pulled up in front of the barbershop where he usually got his hair cut. As Matthew opened the car door, he was nervous and his hands already felt sweaty. He hated getting his hair cut. Everything about it was terrible. The cape the barber put around him felt like it was going to choke him. The sound of the scissors cutting sent chills down his back. Worst of all, he couldn't stand the feeling of loose hairs down his back. Every time he had his hair cut, he immediately wanted to take off his shirt and do something, anything, to stop that itchy feeling. And when the barber was all done, the haircut was usually way too short!

For You to Do

Have you ever had a bad haircut experience? Draw a picture or write a few sentences that describe what made this experience unpleasant.

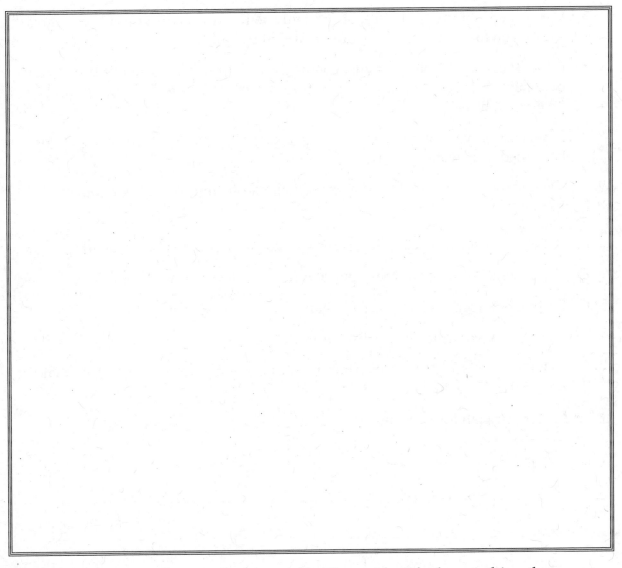

Look back at your picture or what you wrote. Try to identify the one thing that bothered you the most. Write it here:

_____

... And More to Do

Once you know what is bothering you, you can make a plan so future haircuts will be better. Here are some possibilities:

- If it bothers you when the stylist suddenly swings the chair around, you can ask the person to let you know before turning the chair.

- If it bothers you when the stylist combs through your hair, you can brush your own hair so there aren't any tangles. Sometimes it helps to massage your head before you brush.

- If the blow-dryer bothers you, you can ask the stylist to use a towel or let your hair air-dry instead.

We've listed some additional ideas that could help. If one might work for you, put a check mark next to it.

- ☐ Ask the stylist to let you spray your own hair or not to use spray at all.

- ☐ Use earplugs to block out the sound of the scissors.

- ☐ Distract yourself with a handheld game.

- ☐ Bring a clean shirt to change into after the haircut.

- ☐ Ask the stylist to put a towel around your neck with the cape over it, so that hair can't get down your shirt.

Write down your plan for your next haircut.

_____

_____

_____

For You to Know

Keeping yourself looking good and smelling good are important parts of making friends and feeling good about yourself.

Justin glared at his mom. "I'd rather live in Siberia and eat bugs!"

"Well, I'll see if I can get a plane ticket for you later. But right now, you need to take a bath," his mom replied.

Justin hated every part of taking a bath. He hated getting in. It felt like a shock. Once he was finally in the water, it was all right—until the shampoo came. The bubbles felt like ... well, bugs crawling all over him.

Getting out of the tub was the worst. It was so cold! And he hated the feel of the towel rubbing over his body as he tried to get dry. Drying his hair with the towel even hurt.

For You to Do

In the box below, draw a picture or write some words that describe the parts of a bath or shower that you don't usually like.

... And More to Do

How can you make the bad parts of your bath or shower better? We've listed some ideas below to get you thinking.

- Use a shower cap to keep your hair from getting wet.

- Use swim goggles so the soap doesn't get in your eyes.

- Turn on the heat in the room so the air is warm.

- Play some relaxing music. (Make sure that whatever you use to play music is far away from the water.)

- Instead of using a towel, have a parent use a blow-dryer to dry your body.

- Use soap and shampoo that have your favorite smell.

- Instead of getting all the way into a full tub of water, use a little bit of water and a sponge to wash yourself.

- Find ways to have fun—finger paint with different colored soaps, blow bubbles, or sing.

Draw a picture or write some words to describe what could be a good bath or shower.

Once you've come up with some ideas, give them a try!

For You to Do

When was the last time you got upset with your brother or sister? Try to see a picture of this event in your mind and draw it here.

> ## For You to Know
>
> When you understand what your brother or sister does that gets you upset, you can take steps to cope with it when it happens. You can also take steps to prevent it from happening again.

"Mom, Evan's in my room making a mess!" Lauren called. She turned to her brother and said angrily, "Get out of my room!"

But Evan didn't move, so Lauren called louder, "He's going to ruin my work! Mom! Help!"

When her mom came in, fully expecting walls to be torn, furniture destroyed, and carpet ripped apart by this wild thing called Evan, she saw Lauren's brother with a barely detectable smile on his face.

Evan gazed at his mom peacefully, even sweetly, and calmly said, "I didn't do anything." But his face wore a faint, yet satisfied look. Perhaps it was the look of a job well done.

Lauren, however, had puffy, red eyes, welling with tears. Her mom looked back at her with a face of understanding and then turned and looked at her brother. Evan's face dropped.

In one sentence, describe what your brother or sister did that bothered you the most.

_____

Write some words to describe how this made you feel.

_____

What did you do? Did you run away? Cry? Yell? Hit?

_____

What did you do after this event?

_____

What do you think was the purpose of your brother or sister bothering you? Put a check mark next to the choice that you think fits best, or write your own idea on the blank line.

☐ To get attention

☐ For entertainment

☐ To get something from you

☐ To upset you

☐ For no reason—he or she probably didn't mean to bother you.

☐ _____

Your brother or sister may bother you for different reasons. Draw a line from each reason to the solution you think would work best.

If your brother or sister ...

is trying to get attention

wants to be entertained

wants to get something
from you

wants to be left alone

you could ...

tell your parent.

try to respect that desire.

suggest an activity that he or she enjoys, so the focus for entertainment is not on you. If that doesn't work, ask your parent for help.

play a game together or encourage some other way to get attention.

Look back at your picture of when your brother or sister was last bothering you. What was his or her purpose in bothering you?

_____

If this were to happen again, what would you do?

_____

_____

... And More to Do

If your brother or sister is hurting you, tell your parent right away. If he or she drives you crazy now and then, but without really hurting you, you can follow these steps:

- Write down three things you like about your brother or sister.

    1. _____

    2. _____

    3. _____

- Complete this sentence: "It bothers me when you _____
  _____ "

- At a calm moment, ask a parent to sit down with you and your brother or sister. Tell your brother or sister the three things you like, and share a recent memory of a time when you had fun together.

- Share what you wrote about being bothered, and ask your brother or sister to stop that behavior.

For You to Know

It's important to feel comfortable in your classroom. When you feel comfortable, it's easier to get your work done and be successful.

Latisha felt like she was sitting on a stone. Zach sat across from her, making burping noises. She wanted her teacher to help, but his breath bothered her so she didn't want to ask. She looked down at the papers falling out of her desk. "This desk is teeny tiny," she thought, "and there's stuff all over the room, stuff everywhere. I'm going crazy! I feel like I'm trapped."

"How are you doing on your math?" asked her teacher.

"Oh, fine. I've got it," Latisha lied.

She was afraid she'd either start crying or yell if her teacher didn't go away. It was all too much.

Taking Care of Your Senses in the Classroom

For You to Do

There are usually things that kids like about school and things that they wish were different. Write down five things you like about school and five things you don't like.

Things I Like

1. _____

2. _____

3. _____

4. _____

5. _____

Things I Don't Like

1. _____

2. _____

3. _____

4. _____

5. _____

Taking Care of Your Senses in the Classroom

... And More to Do

We've listed some things below that usually help kids' senses in the classroom. Put a check mark next to those things that you think might help. On the blank spaces, write your own ideas to make your classroom better.

☐ A desk that's a comfortable size

☐ Sitting close to the teacher

☐ Things to handle quietly, like a squeeze ball

☐ A seat cushion

☐ Earplugs for quiet work

☐ Quiet space

☐ A rocking chair

☐ Chewing gum

☐ Extra time to complete assignments

☐ A desk that's away from other kids

☐ Soft lights

☐ Taking breaks to move around

☐ A slanted surface for writing

☐ A box to keep your materials in

☐ _____

☐ _____

☐ _____

Talk about these ideas with your parent. Maybe you can come up with even more ways to be comfortable in your class. Together, you can talk with your teacher so that a plan can be made to help you be even more successful at school.

For You to Know

Playing on the playground at recess can be fun, and it can also help you do better in school. After you play hard, you are likely to be more relaxed for the rest of the day.

"I don't understand how to do these problems, Ms. Dunn!" Jayden had been trying to finish his math unit most of the morning, and now he felt irritated.

"Jayden, it's time for recess. I think it will help if you go outside and take a break," Ms. Dunn said.

Jayden ran outside and found his friends playing soccer. He really wanted to score a goal. He ran and ran after the ball, trying to get it away from the other team. Finally, he had it under control and ran down the field. Buzz! The bell rang. Figures, just as he was about to score.

As he lined up for class, Jayden was sweaty but couldn't help but notice how much better he felt. He was smiling and relaxed with his friends. Back in the classroom, he found that the math problems were starting to make sense.

For You to Do

In the space below, draw a picture of what you usually do on the playground.

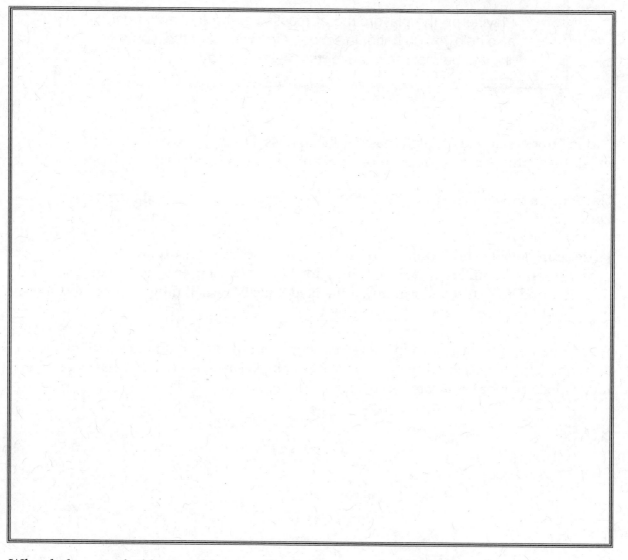

What helps you feel better able to work when you return to class?

_____

_____

_____

... And More to Do

There are many activities that might be fun for you and also help you be better able to focus when you get back to class. From the list that follows, put a check mark next to five that you'd like to try the next time you're out on the playground.

If you think movement would help get you focused, you could

- ☐ throw a ball against a wall and catch it
- ☐ slide
- ☐ swing
- ☐ climb on monkey bars or another play structure
- ☐ jump rope
- ☐ play hopscotch
- ☐ play tag

If you think quieter activities would help you get focused, you could

- ☐ read a book
- ☐ with another kid, take turns hiding small toys in the sand and finding them
- ☐ play a board game or card game
- ☐ do a puzzle
- ☐ look for treasures like interesting rocks or old coins
- ☐ find a cool spot and listen to music

Write down your own ideas to help you get focused.

_____

_____

_____

Help for Handwriting

For You to Know

Handwriting is an important part of school. Some kids with who have trouble with their senses have a hard time with handwriting, but there are tools that can help.

Kai's teacher told him that he had to read his story to the class next. He tried to practice by reading his story to himself, starting at the top of the page, but he could barely read his writing. "What does that word say?" he wondered. He had no idea what he had written.

Kai was really nervous. He figured that he'd probably just make up the story if he couldn't read it. He had worked for two hours on this story the night before. It seemed like it had taken him forever to write, and when it was all done, he couldn't read it. He was sure that his teacher wouldn't be able to read it either.

For You to Do

Look at a recent assignment you've written. Can you read it easily? Ask a friend or family member to read it. Can that person read it easily? On the scale below, rate your handwriting. A score of 0 means that what you wrote is really, really hard to read, or even impossible—like markings from aliens. A score of 10 means that it's clear and perfectly formed, and your teacher would be thrilled.

0　　1　　2　　3　　4　　5　　6　　7　　8　　9　　10

(impossible, or close to it)　　　　　(okay)　　　　　(perfection)

If your handwriting is less than perfect, read the list below of things that may help. Put a check mark next to each choice you'd like to try.

☐ Pencil grips

☐ A weighted pencil

☐ A slanted surface to put your paper on

☐ A plastic writing surface on your desk to keep your paper from moving

☐ Paper with more space between the lines

☐ Paper that has raised lines

☐ Extra time to complete writing tasks

☐ Using a keyboard to type

What other ideas can you think of? Write them here.

_____

_____

_____

Share your ideas with your parent and teacher so they can help get the materials you need. Then try out your ideas for a week. Did your writing get better and easier? If so, which idea helped the most? Write this idea here:

_____

... And More to Do

It may help if your parent, your teacher, and you all meet together. Your parent and teacher might have other ideas too. If everyone thinks it would be appropriate, a plan can be made that lists all the things you need to help you with writing in school. With this plan, it's possible that you can have some of the help you mentioned above when you have to take important tests.

For You to Know

Being comfortable and focused at your work space is important so that you can do your best work.

Brianna sat down at her new desk in the classroom. After about five minutes, her legs started to hurt. She wriggled in her chair to get more comfortable. The chair seemed too big, and the desk too small. She couldn't help but lean way over on her desk. Her back started hurting. She wriggled some more. Arggh! She was so uncomfortable.

Her teacher noticed her squirming, trying to find some comfort.

"Oh, Brianna, we need to adjust your desk and chair. Your feet should be flat on the floor, and your elbows should rest comfortably."

After her teacher had finished adjusting, Brianna sat down again. She actually felt pretty comfortable! "A pillow on my seat would help even more," she thought.

For You to Do

Read this list of ways to make your work space at school comfortable so that you can focus and learn more easily. Place a check mark next to each strategy you'd like to talk over with your teacher and parent. Write your own ideas on the blank lines.

- Earplugs

- A cushion for your chair

- Chewing gum or a straw

- A desk and chair that fit you well

- A weighted vest

- A desk away from distractions

- A timer or clock on your desk

- Pencil grips

- A slanted surface to write on

- Paper with raised lines or more space between lines

- A keyboard

- Having a crunchy or chewy snack available

- Containers for your supplies to keep things organized

- _____

- _____

- _____

... And More to Do

From the items you just checked, choose three ideas that you'd like to talk with your parent and teacher about, and write them below. These ideas should be the ones that you think can best help you stay calm and focused while you do your work.

1. _____

2. _____

3. _____

For You to Know

There are lots of ways to stay organized. Knowing that you can find your stuff will help you feel more relaxed and calm.

"Mom, where's my homework!" Ethan called. His voice sounded upset.

"Ethan, the bus is going to come in exactly three minutes. Why aren't you ready?" his mom responded.

"Mom, I have to find my homework. If I don't, I can't have bonus recess!"

Ethan began to panic. He couldn't think. Where was his homework! He felt like he was about to cry. The bus would be coming soon.

His mom came to his door. "Ethan, you don't even have your shoes on!"

Ethan looked down. She was right. Where were his shoes! So much for his homework. He didn't have time to look any longer. Even though it was going to be a beautiful sunny day, he grabbed what was in front of him—snow boots that were still out from a month ago when it last snowed. At least they were easy to get on.

As he boarded the bus, his friend asked, "Ethan, why are you wearing snow boots?"

For You to Do

Put a check mark next to each of the following strategies for keeping organized that you'd be willing to try. Use the blank lines to add your own ideas.

- ☐ Planning ahead
- ☐ Keeping your work space clean
- ☐ Following a schedule
- ☐ Writing down things to remember
- ☐ Putting things back where you found them
- ☐ Using a timer, watch, or clock to keep track of time
- ☐ Recycling things you don't use
- ☐ Storing materials in containers
- ☐ Cleaning out your backpack and desk every day

☐ _____

☐ _____

☐ _____

... And More to Do

What are your three most prized possessions? List them here:

1. _____

2. _____

3. _____

Next to each, write down where you think it is. Now check to see if those possessions are where you think they are.

If they are not, write one way to keep organized that you'd be willing to focus on for the next week.

_____

_____

If they are, congratulations! Do you think you can be even more organized? If so, write down one strategy that you'd like to try.

_____

_____

Identifying Your Strengths

For You to Know

Knowing and focusing on your strengths can help you feel better about yourself. And if your parent and teacher are aware of your strengths, they can help you be even more successful.

Carlos was feeling frustrated. It had taken him forever to read all the pages he was supposed to read for homework. Even after he read everything, he didn't really understand what was happening in the book. Carlos felt like he wasn't good at anything.

As he approached the door to his classroom, his friend Chad came up to him and asked, "Carlos, can you help me with problem five on the math homework?"

"Oh, that one was easy," Carlos replied, and he explained how to solve it.

"Thanks! I couldn't figure that one out. It was starting to drive me crazy," Chad said.

Later, Julia came up to his desk and asked, "Carlos, can you draw a horse for our project? I'm working on the summary and wanted to include a picture."

As Carlos finished drawing a horse, which did look good, he thought that maybe there were some things he did well—just not reading.

For You to Do

Think of your school day. What are you good at? It might help to think of things that are generally easy for you or things that people ask you to help with. Maybe you are good at drawing, reading, multiplying, or playing soccer.

Write down five things you are good at in school.

1. _____

2. _____

3. _____

4. _____

5. _____

Now think of your time away from school. What do you do well at home or during the weekends? Maybe you set the table well, or maybe you are good at riding your bike, fishing, singing, or dancing. You might also be good with animals, or you might be a helpful brother or sister. Maybe you listen well to your parent! That's a great thing to be good at.

Write down five strengths you have at home.

1. _____

2. _____

3. _____

4. _____

5. _____

... And More to Do

Look back at your two lists. Tell how you feel about yourself when you read them.

_____

_____

_____

Be sure to share your list of strengths with your parent and your teacher. They might be able to help you use your strengths to do well at other things. Or they might be able to plan activities that build on your strengths so you have fun while learning or being at home.

For You to Know

Your teacher is the first person to go to if you or your parent thinks you need additional support at school. There may also be other people at your school who can help. It will be easier for your teacher and others to help you if they know what you are good at and what is hard for you.

Although Olivia was in fourth grade, she couldn't really read. She was terrified of being asked to read something out loud in class. But when her teacher, Ms. Miller, read her a story, Olivia could follow everything. It was like she could make a movie in her head and go back and watch it over and over again. She even remembered stories that were read to her in first grade. Why couldn't everything be read to her?

When she was alone with Ms. Miller, struggling through a sentence in a "baby" book, she asked, "Is there a way that I can have books read to me? I remember everything that I hear. I just can't read books the way other kids do."

Ms. Miller looked at Olivia and said, "You know Olivia, I think that's a good suggestion. We still need to work on having you read yourself, but I think we should talk more with you and your parents about this idea."

For You to Do

It's important that people who want to help you keep in mind your strengths, instead of focusing only on things that you have a hard time with. Your teacher and others at school can use your strengths to help you with things that are hard. For example, if you're good at using the computer, your teacher can have you use that to write instead of using a pencil and paper. Read each of the following and put a check mark next to those things that are strengths for you.

☐ Are you good at focusing on things that you need to do?

☐ Are you good at writing with a pencil?

☐ Are you able to ask for help when you need it?

☐ Do you share ideas and ask questions during discussion?

☐ Are you good at physical games like soccer, or throwing and catching a ball?

☐ Are you good at reading?

☐ Are you good at writing?

☐ Are you good at math?

☐ Are you good at using computers?

☐ Are you good at drawing?

☐ Are you good at putting things together with your hands?

☐ Are you good at music?

What else would you tell your teacher that you are good at?

_____

_____

_____

... And More to Do

To understand how to help you, your teacher might want to know about some things that are often hard for kids who have trouble with their senses. Read each of the following, and put a check mark next to those things that are difficult for you.

- ☐ Sitting at your desk

- ☐ Distractions, like people talking or moving

- ☐ Having people get too close to you or touch you

- ☐ Physical activities, like baseball or basketball

- ☐ Handwriting

- ☐ Keeping things organized

Are there any other areas where you think you need more help? If so, what are they?

_____

_____

_____

Why do you think you need more help for these areas?

_____

_____

_____

For You to Know

Smiling, saying hello, and being relaxed are great first steps to making friends. Being around friends can help you learn new things, have fun, and be happier!

Haley watched as her teacher came toward her with the new girl in her class. They were talking and smiling, and Haley was somewhat surprised at how relaxed the girl seemed. When they reached Haley, the girl smiled and said, "Hi, I'm Courtney. What's your name?"

After a second, Haley replied, "I'm Haley."

"Well, it's nice to meet you! I hope you can show me around at recess. I don't know anyone here, but I'm looking forward to making some new friends," said Courtney. The whole time she spoke, she was smiling. She seemed so positive. Haley felt good being around her.

For You to Do

Why do you think Haley felt good about being around Courtney?

_____

_____

What did Courtney do or say to indicate that she wanted to be friends with Haley? Write three clues here:

1. _____

2. _____

3. _____

Think of a time when you wanted to be friends with someone. How did you let that person know?

_____

_____

... And More to Do

What have you seen other kids do or say that makes them seem like they would be good friends to have?

_____

_____

_____

What do you do or say to let other kids know that you would be a good friend?

_____

_____

_____

Are there people at school that you'd like to be friends with? If so, write down their names, and tell when and how you will let them know.

_____

_____

_____

Activity 35

Finding People to Help You

For You to Know

You are not alone. There are lots of people, both kids and adults, who want to help if and when you need it.

Cody was sitting at his desk, trying to figure out how to do a math problem. He tried to make a drawing to help him solve the problem, but his drawing just looked like circles that had been sat on. He erased what he had drawn. He tried drawing a number line, but that didn't help. He erased his work again. Next, Cody looked around to see if there were clues on any of the posters that hung in the room. All he saw was a spider on the wall. He didn't say anything; he liked spiders.

Cody sighed and looked at his paper. It looked like it had been run through a machine to erase pencil markings again and again, and then gotten stuck.

"Do you need some help?" asked Caleb, who sat across from him.

"Yes, I think I do," Cody replied gratefully.

For You to Do

Draw a line from each problem to the person you would go to for help. There might be more than one person who can help with each problem.

You can't figure out a math problem.	Police officer
An older student is trying to get your backpack.	Classmate
Another kid is calling you names.	Teacher
You see someone walking with a knife.	Principal
You're at school and forgot your lunch money.	Parent
You usually feel frustrated at school.	Any adult

... And More to Do

Describe the last time you needed help.

_____

_____

_____

Whom did you go to for help?

_____

Did you get the help you needed? Tell what happened.

_____

_____

_____

Whom else could you have gone to?

_____

For You to Know

At one time or another, all people have days when they've done something they're sorry for. You can learn from these mistakes to make yourself a better person, feel good about yourself, and make tomorrow great!

Sitting in the principal's office, Bella felt terrible. She was so afraid of how her parents were going to react when they got the call from the principal.

"I didn't mean to hit Luke," Bella said. The principal looked like he didn't believe her.

"Okay, I hit Luke and I shouldn't have." There. She had said it.

She had hit Luke in her class. He had made her so angry! They were working together on their reading assignment, and he kept scratching his nails on his jacket. It made the worst sound! It drove her crazy! She had asked him to stop, and he didn't. She had tried to ignore him, but he kept making that awful sound. She was already upset by the noise, and when Luke called her stupid because she couldn't read well, she lost it.

For You to Do

Have you ever done something you were sorry for? Draw a picture in the space below to show what happened.

Were one or more of your senses (touch, taste, smell, hearing, or sight) part of the problem? If so, describe how.

_____

_____

_____

... And More to Do

How did you feel about yourself after your bad day?

_____

_____

What did you learn from your mistake?

_____

_____

What did you do, or could you have done, to make the situation better?

_____

_____

Tell about any part of this situation that you think you handled well.

_____

_____

What is one thing you would do differently if a situation like this happens again?

_____

_____

For You to Know

Bullying is a serious problem, but there are ways to reduce the chances of being a target for bullies. If you are being bullied, you need to inform your parent, teacher, or principal. It's just as important to get help if you see someone else being bullied.

Patricia was standing by the school doorway, looking to see where her friends were on the playground. She noticed Rebecca sitting alone on one of the benches. Rebecca wasn't one of her friends, but Patricia felt sorry for her. Her hair was always a mess, and she was always dropping things. She never seemed to talk to anyone. It seemed like just about everyone teased Rebecca about something.

"Hi, Rebecca …" called Samantha from across the playground. She was heading toward the bench where Rebecca sat.

"Oh no!" Patricia thought. This wasn't going to be good. Samantha was mean. She traveled with a pack of three other girls who liked to do whatever they could to make kids like Rebecca cry.

Patricia quickly gathered a few other kids and said, "If we go sit with Rebecca, maybe Samantha will back off. If that doesn't work, we can ask a teacher to help."

For You to Do

Read these passages and rank who you think a bully would pick on first, second, and third. Write the number next to each passage.

_____ Lots of kids liked Zack. He was always smiling and was just fun to be around. At recess, he was usually playing a game with other kids. All the teachers seemed to know him too.

_____ Lucy dressed nicely and looked like she fit in with everyone else. At recess, she usually hung out with one other girl, drawing at a table or playing in the sand. She was really quiet, but she never looked sad. In fact, she always looked relaxed and calm.

_____ Mark always wore the same clothes and never seemed to take a bath. He smelled. When kids teased him, he would start to cry. He didn't seem to have any friends.

Write the name of the child you think a bully would pick on first.

_____

Tell why you think this.

_____

_____

... *And More to Do*

If you have ever been the victim of a bully, tell what happened.

_____

_____

How did you handle it?

_____

_____

If you've never been a victim of a bully, what would you do if you were?

_____

_____

Talk over your answers with your parent.

Making Sense of Your Senses

Helping Other Kids

For You to Know

Helping other kids who might also be struggling with their senses is a great way make friends, earn respect from others, and feel good about yourself.

Over the weekend, Carissa's teacher had rearranged all the desks in the classroom. Carissa gathered her stuff from her old spot and went over to sit at her new desk, next to her new partner, Melanie. As Carissa was putting things neatly into her desk, she couldn't help noticing that Melanie's books and papers were falling out onto the floor. Melanie picked up a paper, put it back into her desk, and then another paper fell out. It was a mess.

When it came time to write, Melanie practically lay on top of her desk. She gripped her pencil with five fingers and pressed hard as she wrote. When she was only one sentence into her assignment, her paper ripped.

Later in the day, Melanie complained that her back and feet hurt. "Here's what I do. Maybe it will help you," said Carissa. "I put my jacket behind my back when I work. It feels like a pillow, and it helps me sit up straight. I also put a book under my feet when I work. My feet feel better, and the book also helps me sit up."

"Sounds good," replied Melanie. "I'll try that."

"I can also help you clean out your desk, if you'd like," Carissa added.

"I appreciate that—maybe tomorrow. It might take all day!" Melanie smiled.

For You to Do

You might have, or have had, someone in your class who has difficulty with

- Sitting up
- Keeping organized
- Eating different foods
- Coping with noise, smells, or bright lights
- Things touching them

Tell what this person had difficulty with.

_____

_____

How could you tell that this person was having difficulty?

_____

_____

Were there ways that you could have helped? Tell how.

_____

_____

How do you think this person would have reacted if you had offered help?

_____

_____

... And More to Do

Why do you think it's important to help other people?

_____

_____

_____

_____

_____

For You to Know

You can achieve incredible things in your life by believing in yourself and setting goals along the way to get to where you want to go.

"What do you want to do when you grow up?" Morgan asked.

"I think it would be fun to be a pilot," replied her friend Amanda. "I love the feeling when a plane takes off. The last time we went on a plane, I laughed when the engines roared and the plane started to race along the runway. It's got to be the coolest thing in the world."

"That does sound like fun," Morgan said.

"And I'd get to travel all over and see new places," Amanda added. "Plus, I just think I'd like flying. I love looking at the clouds and the sky from a plane way up in the air. It's peaceful."

For You to Do

Create a picture of yourself as an adult. If you'd like, you can paint, draw, write, or make a collage with magazine pictures. Be sure to include what you'd like to be doing and where you'd like to live. Add any other detail you'd like to make it really clear what your vision is for yourself. This picture is for you.

... And More to Do

What are some steps you need to take in order to achieve your vision? Put a star next to the one you think is most important.

_____

_____

Write down what you would need to do in order to take your most important step. For example, if your most important step is to learn how to fly, you might make this list: find out about flight-training schools, learn how airplanes work, or (with your parent's help) talk to a pilot.

_____

_____

Choose one of these steps that you'd like to focus on. Write it here:

_____

Now set a goal to achieve this step. A goal generally has two parts—what and when.

What are you going to do?

_____

By when will you do it?

_____

For You to Know

You've worked hard and learned a lot—about yourself, your senses, and about the world around you. Having difficulty with your senses certainly isn't easy, but we think the challenges you've overcome and the lessons you've learned will make you a stronger person. For that, you deserve to celebrate.

Brandon closed the book and put it down on the table. He felt proud to have done so much work. "I feel better talking to my teacher about what I need to do well in school," he thought. "I also know how to keep myself comfortable and calm."

He decided he deserved a reward for his efforts. He thought a bit and then asked his mom if he could have a friend spend the night. They would watch a movie and have some ice cream.

For You to Do

Make yourself a certificate of achievement. The certificate is for you and about you, so make it any way you'd like.

Making Sense of Your Senses

... And More to Do

It's time to celebrate! There are lots of fun ways to celebrate. Maybe you'd like to have a friend over for a treat. Or maybe you'd like to do something special with your parent, like going shopping for a new game. There's also the BIG reward that you listed under Activity 1.

What will you do to celebrate?

_____

_____

_____

_____

_____

Christopher R. Auer, MA, is the disabilities and mental health administrator for the Head Start program in the Denver Mayor's Office for Education and Children. He is also affiliate faculty at Regis University and coauthor of Parenting a Child with Sensory Processing Disorder. He is a regular presenter at national conferences.

Michelle M. Auer, MS, OTR, is an occupational therapist for a school district in the Denver area. She also maintains a private practice providing hippotherapy for children.